THE DENTAL PRESCRIBER

by

Dr. Colin B. Lessell

MB, BS (Lond), BDS (Lond), MRCS (Eng), LRCP (Lond)

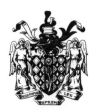

THE BRITISH HOMOEOPATHIC ASSOCIATION

27a Devonshire Street

London, W1N 1RJ

INDEX

WHAT IS HOMOEOPATHY?

HOMOEOPATHY is a branch of medicine which necessitates a competent knowledge of all other subjects included in the term *"medicine"* — anatomy, physiology, pathology, bacteriology, biochemistry, psychiatry and clinical diagnosis. But before detectable pathological changes appear, a patient often has symptoms, and the homoeopath in treating these early stages of disease, saves his patient more often than he knows from serious illness.

Homoeopathy has discovered that substances which are poisonous in their natural state can be used to cure, but to cure only that which they can cause. The name HOMOEOPATHY — from the Greek *"homoios"* (similar) and *"pathos"* (suffering) — expresses its basic principle — *"the curing of likes by likes"*.

The use of minute doses is a necessary corollary of this principle. Indeed, the great power of the infinitely little, and the opposite effect of large and small doses have been demonstrated in recent times in connection with vitamins, the minute traces of certain minerals necessary to plant life, and atomic fission.

Homoeopathic remedies are derived from all the kingdoms of nature, including such varied substances as bee stings and snake venoms, arsenic, gold and silica (sand) and even from disease tissues. To date, upwards of 2,000 different such medicines are known, although a much smaller number is found adequate for common use. In fact, about 24 would form the basis of a domestic medicine chest. Twelve will suffice for a first-aid outfit.

Each remedy has different characteristics which demand individual treatment to prepare the initial, or "mother" tincture (ø). Having reached this stage, the pharmacist can undertake the potentisation.

Whilst it must be emphasised that the practice of Homoeopathy entails a detailed knowledge of the *materia medica,* nevertheless, first-aid and other emergencies can often be treated homoeopathically with eminently satisfactory results. This is partly because of the "affinities" of various remedies for particular tissues, and because experience has shown that injuries and common ailments usually respond to certain well-proved remedies.

Relief may be obtained in the case of accidents such as burns, bruises, cuts and stings. And ailments such as coughs, colds, sore throats and indigestion may be alleviated without danger of the undesirable after-effects which so often follow the indiscriminate use of the commonly prescribed drugs.

The doses recommended are so minute that, provided they are not repeated too frequently or over too long a period, they will not do harm. But whatever the trouble, it must be most strongly stressed that if any of these conditions do not readily yield to treatment, professional aid should be sought.

Taken from *"A Guide to HOMOEOPATHY, Rational Medicine",*
published by The British Homoeopathic Association,
27a Devonshire Street, London, W1N 1RJ.

INTRODUCTION

The Dental Prescriber is intended for the use of the general dental practitioner, the dental specialist, and the homoeopathically orientated patient. It must be emphasised that the remedial measures suggested herein are not intended to replace the *mechanical* arts of modern Dentistry, but are to be regarded as highly useful and effective complements. Only inasmuch as they replace, and indeed surpass, the use of *drugs,* such as antibiotics, are they in contravention of the dicta of the pundits.

With regard to remedies, there are two scales of potency quoted in the text: the decimal (number of serial dilutions, followed by suffix "x"), and the centesimal (number of serial dilutions, *no* suffix attached). The symbol "ø" denotes undiluted mother tincture. The decimal scale involves serial dilution of 1/10, and the centesimal, serial dilution of 1/100. Hence, 6x corresponds to a dilution of $1/10^6$ (one part per million), and 6 corresponds to a dilution of $1/10^{12}$ (one part per billion). The most commonly used potencies are 6 and 30.

The text is arranged alphabetically, with adequate cross-reference between specialist terms and those of common parlance. After each rubric, a number of remedies is generally quoted. These are to be regarded as alternatives in most instances, for it is usually better to prescribe a single remedy at one time. Where the differentiation between the remedies is straightforward, the differentiating factors are given. Where the differentiation is either complex or difficult, the remedies are simply listed without qualification. In these instances, the reader is advised to consult a standard work of homoeopathic *materia medica,* lest he/she be committed to trial and error. There are, however, many exceptions to the rule of the single remedy, and it will be noted that the text specifies the use of combinations or alternations of remedies in special circumstances. Certainly, even if not stated, topical (local) treatments can always be combined with systemic remedial therapy. All the remedies listed are to be systemically administered, unless it is specifically stated that they are for topical use.

Systemic administration (dispersion through the body) involves dissolving the remedy either on or under the tongue, from which site the remedy is rapidly absorbed. The systemic remedy may be supplied as drops, or in the form of tablets or spherical pilules. For small children, unconscious or semiconscious patients, they are best administered as drops or powders (which may be pulverised tablets/pilules). The dosage for adults and children is the same; a single dose being three drops, one pilule, or one tablet. Reinforcement of action is not effected by increasing the material quantity of the dose. This is achieved either by using a higher potency (greater dilution), or by dose repetition at intervals. Throughout the text, I have taken the liberty of suggesting potency and probable interval between doses. These matters are not, however, inflexible. They will serve as a useful guide to the new prescriber, and in the light of his/her developing experience, he/she must feel free to modify them.

Remedies should always be stocked by the dental surgeon himself for use in emergencies, and the same remedies deserve a place in the domestic chest. These are readily obtained from distributing homoeopathic pharmacies. All remedies should be protected from daylight, perfumes, other aromatic substances, and unnecessary handling. In general, the consumption of food or drink, and the cleaning of teeth is proscribed within fifteen minutes of taking a systemic remedy. Similarly, the use of mouthwashes should be avoided in this time interval. All forms of coffee (including the decaffeinated variety) should be avoided during a course of remedial therapy. Stored in a cool place, in tightly stoppered bottles, the shelf-life of the remedy is many years.

Finally, remember that there is an overlap of action of remedies. Even if what appears to be the most appropriate remedy is not readily available, you may choose the next most appropriate remedy that is at hand. Much good work can be done in this way. Always discontinue medication once significant improvement has been achieved.

MAJOR REMEDIES

The following is a list of useful remedies to be stocked by the dental surgeon. All are mentioned in the text, and all should be stocked as pilules/tablets, except where otherwise stated. Those marked by an asterisk (*) are the most important basic remedies to be stocked, either by the dental surgeon, or the domestic prescriber.

Acid. nitricum 30
*Apis mellifica 30
Argentum nitricum 30
*Arnica 30 & 200
Baptisia 30
*Belladonna 30
Borax 30
*Calendula ø (drops)
*Calendula (5% cream)
*Carbo veg. 30 (drops)
Chamomilla 30 & 200
Coffea cruda 30
Euphrasia 30
Euphrasia ø (drops)
*Ferrum phos. 30
Gelsemium 30
*Hepar sulph. 6
*Hypericum 30

*Ipecacuanha 30
Lachesis 30
*Ledum 30
*Mercurius sol. 6 & 30
*Myristica 3x
Natrum mur. 30
*Phosphorus 30
*Plantago 6 & *Plantago ø (drops)
*Pyrogen 30
*Rescue Remedy (drops)
Rhus tox. 30
Ruta 6
*Salvia offic. (sage leaves)
Sanguinaria 200
Sepia 6
Silicea 6
Spigelia 200
Staphysagria 30

Other remedies are mentioned throughout the text, and may be added at leisure to the basic stock.

8

THERAPEUTIC INDEX

ABRASION

Frequently at corners of mouth, from instrumentation or manipulation. Apply *Calendula* 5% cream sparingly, thrice daily.

ABSCESS, dental

(1) Initial formative stage, with little swelling, but much throbbing, redness, *Belladonna* 30, ½-hourly.

(2) With foul breath, excessive salivation, *Mercurius sol.* 6, hourly.

(3) In later stage, where frank pus has formed, to encourage it to point and discharge, *Hepar sulph.* 6, 2-hourly.

(4) Where surgical incision would seem essential, *Myristica* 3x, given hourly, may replace the scalpel.

(5) After pus has discharged, to hasten resolution, and removal of loculated pus, *Silicea* 6, twice daily.

(6) Locally, mouthwashes of infusion of *Salvia offic.* (see MOUTHWASHES), hourly.

ANGULAR CHEILITIS (cracked corners of mouth)

Correct overclosure of dentures, and treat as for ABRASION. May be caused by Vitamin B2 (riboflavine) deficiency, in which case replacement therapy is required.

ANTIBIOTICS, ill-effects of

By disturbing the balance of normal flora, systemic disturbance often arises from the use of antibiotics. This problem is avoided by the judicious use of homoeopathic remedies. Where the problem has arisen:

(1) In general, one small carton of yoghurt (goat's yoghurt in those allergic to cow's milk) daily, plus garlic capsules/tablets, 2 morning and evening for an adult (half dose for a child), swallowed with cold water. Garlic and parsley capsules produce less odour, and odourless garlic tablets are available, but are believed to be less effective. Children may nibble garlic tablets, if they are unable to swallow them.

(2) Where diarrhoea has been induced, add *Acidum nitricum* 30, 4-hourly.

(3) Where thrush (oral or vaginal) has been caused, add *Borax* 30, thrice daily. See also THRUSH, oral.

APHTHOUS ULCERS

(1) Locally, mouthwashes of *Salvia offic.* infusion, or *Hydrastis* lotion (see MOUTHWASHES), several times daily.

(2) In nervous patients, very sensitive to loud noises, *Borax* 30, 4-hourly.

(3) Foul breath, tongue large and retains imprint of teeth, *Mercurius sol.* 30, 4-hourly.

(4) Tongue shows imprint of teeth, saliva thick, and tenacious, breath inoffensive, *Hydrastis* 30, 4-hourly.

(5) Ulcers with yellow or yellow-green bases, uvula swollen, *Kali bich.* 30, 4-hourly.

(6) Base of ulcer bleeds, splinter-like or sticking pains, *Acidum nitricum* 30, 4-hourly.

(7) In alcoholics and lactating women, *Acidum sulphuricum* 30, 4-hourly.

(8) Where ulcers do not respond to these simple measures, or where they are recurrent, referral to a homoeopathic physician for constitutional (general) treatment is advised. Intermittent treatment with deep-acting remedies, such as *Sulphur* 30 (to be used with caution/supervision in eczema cases), is often required.

APPREHENSION of patients

(1) Trepidation, diarrhoea, drowsiness, feeling of weakness ("at knees"), loss of memory (largely *hypo*kinetic picture), *Gelsemium* 30, given morning and evening prior to procedure, and one hour before procedure.

(2) Trepidation, diarrhoea, agitation, hurried actions, incessant speech (largely *hyper*kinetic picture), *Argentum nitricum* 30, given morning and evening prior to procedure, and one hour before procedure. (See also CHILDREN, fractious).

BLEEDING

See HAEMATOMA; HAEMORRHAGE, dental; GINGIVITIS, acute ulcerative; PERIODONTITIS, chronic.

BREATH, offensive or foul - See HALITOSIS.

BRUXISM, BRUXOMANIA (Tooth-grinding/clenching)

Bruxism occurs during sleep, whilst bruxomania occurs in the waking hours.

(1) Child grinds teeth whilst asleep with jumping and jerking, ugly and cross nature, dislikes being touched, intestinal worms may be present, *Cina* 30, one hour before retiring.

(2) In overworked business people, with a tendency to over-indulgence and recurrent gastric disturbances, *Nux vomica* 30, twice daily.

(3) In tense, hyperanxious people, inability to relax, highly strung, perfection-istic, inclined to tackle too many jobs at the same time, *Vervain* (Bach), 3 drops thrice daily in a wineglassful of water.

(4) Abandoning the use of coffee in those who are sensitive to its actions, or drink it to great excess, will reduce tension.

(5) In those who crave sweet things, become ravenously hungry and irritable if meals are delayed, shake with hunger, sweat excessively, a diet low in sugars (except in the form of fruit), and refined carbohydrates ("hypoglycaemic diet") may be of assistance.

(6) Vitamin B6 (pyridoxine) in material doses, 50 mg. twice daily, may be

helfpul in some adult cases, especially if they suffer from premenstrual tension, or take the contraceptive pill.

BURNS, instrument
(1) Apply *Calendula* 5% cream sparingly, thrice daily.
(2) Apply the contents of a Vitamin E capsule sparingly, thrice daily.

CALCULUS, dental (Tartar)
To remove tartar from the teeth, or retard its formation:
(1) *Calcarea renalis* 6, twice daily.
(2) *Fragaria* 6, twice daily. (See also SCALING & POLISHING, sore gums after).

CALCULUS, salivary (Salivary gland/duct stone)
Where a stone cannot be removed by simply surgery, there are multiple stones, or there is a general predisposition to stone formation (eg, renal calculi), then homoeopathic therapy is indicated.
(1) *Calcarea renalis* 6, twice daily.
(2) Complement with *Calcarea carbonica* 30, single doses twice weekly (eg, Monday and Fridays).

CANCER, oral - See TUMOURS & CYSTS.

CANCRUM ORIS - See NOMA.

CARIES, predisposition to dental
This may be reduced by appropriate homoeopathic therapy.
(1) In short, squat patients, with a tendency to obesity, flat palate, white square anterior teeth, wide dental arches, absence of crowding, *Calcarea carbonica* 30, single doses twice weekly (eg, Mondays and Fridays).
(2) In tall, thin patients, with a tendency to be hunched, narrow face, well-arched palate, yellowish anterior teeth, rectangular in vertical direction, tendency to crowding, *Calcarea phosphorica* 30, single doses twice weekly.
(3) In patients with obvious asymmetry of face and dental arches, scoliosis of spine, very flexible joints, tendency to recurrent sprains and dislocations, tendency to exostoses, anterior teeth crowded, with poor, grey enamel, *Calcarea fluorica* 30, single doses twice weekly.
(4) Early and rapid decay of deciduous dentition (milk teeth), *Kreosotum* 30, single doses twice weekly.
(5) In conjunction with basic therapy, add *Bacillinum* 30, single doses each month (to be used with caution/supervision in asthmatic cases).
(6) See DIET.

CELLULITIS (Spreading infection of connective tissues)
(1) Reactive oedema of facial tissues, patient thirstless, face feels sore and bruised, *Apis mellifica* 30, 2-hourly.

11

(2) Facial tissues red and tense, throbbing pain, great thirst, *Belladonna* 30, 2-hourly.

(3) Facial tissues become dark bluish or purplish, *Lachesis* 30, 2-hourly.

(4) Where septicaemia threatens, add *Pyrogen* 30, 2-hourly. THIS MAY BE A MOST SERIOUS CONDITION, AND A DENTAL SURGEON/PHYSICIAN MUST BE CONSULTED.

CHILDREN, fractious

(1) Whining restlessness, spiteful, oversensitivity to pain, cross, irritable desire to be carried or petted (which improves), uncooperative, *Chamomilla* 30, morning and evening prior to procedure, and one hour before procedure.

(2) Similar to the former, but does not want to be touched, carried, or even looked at, *Cina* 30, dose repetition as above.

COFFEE, ill-effects of

In addition to causing increased tension in susceptible individuals (see BRUXISM, BRUXOMANIA), coffee is a great antidote to many (though not all) homoeopathic remedies. Its consumption should, therefore, be proscribed during remedial therapy.

COLD-SORE - See HERPES LABIALIS.

COLLAPSE, sudden

Sudden collapse in the surgery calls for mechanical resuscitative techniques, and the availability of Oxygen. Whether the patient has incurred a simple vasovagal attack (simple faint), or something more serious, such as myocardial infarction (heart attack), these measures should be complemented by the oral administration of remedies. These may aid recovery and save life.

(1) In all cases, *Rescue Remedy* (Bach), 3 drops every 2 minutes until recovery occurs.

(2) Additionally, in all cases, *Carbo veg.* 30, a single dose (preferably 3 drops of liquid potency; otherwise, one finely pulverised tablet/pilule).

CONCUSSION, facial fracture with

Where concussion complicates traumatic cases, *Natrum sulph.* 30, 4-hourly, in addition to other remedies indicated. (See FRACTURE, jaw).

CONJUNCTIVITIS of dentists, acute

This may follow contact of the eye with septic particles.

(1) Locally, *Euphrasia* lotion (5-10 drops ø in 1 fl. oz./28 ml. water) as an eyewash, 2-hourly.

(2) Additionally, *Euphrasia* 30, thrice daily.

CYST - See RANULA; TUMOURS & CYSTS.

DECAY, dental - See CARIES, predisposition to dental.

DENTURE, ill-fitting
Sore mouth and ulceration due to ill-fitting/over-extended denture:
(1) Locally, mouthwashes of *Salvia offic.* infusion or *Calendula* lotion (see MOUTHWASHES), several times daily.
(2) *Arnica* 30, thrice daily.

DERMATITIS of dentists - See ECZEMA of dentists.

DIET
(1) For the preservation of general health, as well as that of the oral tissues, a good diet should have the following features:
   absence of refined carbohydrates
   low salt content (more will be required by those who live or work in hot environments)
   low animal fats
   generous supply of whole grains
   fresh fruit, fresh vegetables (a good quantity to be eaten raw)
   absence of artificial colouring and preservatives
(2) Where recurrent gastric problems (hyperacidity, dyspepsia, indigestion, ulcer, etc.) are associated with a high caries predisposition, and crumbling of teeth, the patient should consume raw, grated cabbage (green, white or red) on a daily basis, plus fresh alfalfa, when available. Alternatively, compressed alfalfa tablets, 2 after meals, thrice daily.
(3) Whereas the addition of fluoride to the drinking water reduces the incidence of caries, it is not without risk to those of a "fluoric constitution". These are persons of asymmetrical development, with lax ligaments, tendency to scoliosis, sprains, and the formation of exostoses. Acromegaly constitutes a variant of the fluoric constitution. Such people are highly susceptible to the toxic effects of fluoride, and should not drink fluoridated water. (See CARIES, predisposition to dental).

DRY SOCKET (Infected socket)
(1) Locally, mouthwashes of *Salvia offic.* infusion (see MOUTHWASHES), several times daily.
(2) Throbbing pain, *Belladonna* 30, hourly.
(3) Pain unbearable, tosses in anguish, relieved by holding cold water in mouth, *Coffea cruda* 30, $\frac{1}{4}$-hourly.
(4) To promote resolution thereafter, *Hepar* 6, 4-hourly.
(5) To speed the expulsion of sequestra, *Silicea* 6, twice daily.
(6) Locally, dressings impregnated with *Plantago* ø.

ECZEMA of dentists
The occurrence of eczema on the hands of the operator will usually require the latter to consult a homoeopathic physician. However, immediate measures include:

13

(1) Locally, to control itching, *Viola tricolor* (10 drops ø to 1 fl. oz./28 ml. water), applied sparingly as necessary.

(2) Locally, to treat cracking and weeping, *Graphites* 8x cream, applied sparingly, 2-hourly.

EPISTAXIS, acute (Nosebleed)
(1) This is usually controllable with *Ferrum phos.* 30, ½-hourly.

(2) Additionally, where the patient is very distressed, *Rescue Remedy* (Bach), 3 drops ¼-hourly.

ERUPTION of teeth, delayed
Especially in podgy children, *Calcarea carbonica* 30, twice weekly (eg, Mondays and Fridays).

ERUPTION, painful - See TEETHING, constitutional upsets in.

EYE-STRAIN of dentists
Ruta 6, hourly.

FAINT - See COLLAPSE, sudden.

FEAR of dentistry - See APPREHENSION of patients; CHILDREN, fractious; & PAIN THRESHOLD, low.

FISTULA, oro-antral
(1) *Acidum fluoricum* 6, twice daily.

(2) Should this fail, then *Silicea* 6, twice daily.

FLUORIDATION of water - See DIET.

FRACTURE, jaw
(1) To relieve pains of fractured bones, *Rhus tox.* 30 and *Bryonia* 30, in 2-hourly alternation.

(2) To relieve pain, when bones are severely contused, *Ruta* 30, 2-hourly.

(3) To promote sleep after injury, add *Sticta pulmonaria* 200, as required.

(4) To promote union, *Symphytum* 3x, thrice daily.

(5) Additionally, to promote union, *Calcarea carbonica* 30, single doses twice weekly (eg, Mondays and Fridays).

(6) Additionally, for bruising of soft tissues, *Arnica* 30, thrice daily.

(7) For delayed or non-union, *Ruta* 6, twice daily.

(8) For stiffness in mobilising phase, *Ruta* 6 and *Rhus tox.* 30, in 4-hourly alternation.

(9) To encourage the regeneration of damaged nerves, add *Hypericum* 6, twice daily. (See also CONCUSSION, facial fracture with; & HAEMATOMA.)

GINGIVITIS, acute ulcerative (Vincent's stomatitis)
(1) With heavily coated tongue, *Mercurius sol.* 30, thrice daily.
(2) With clean tongue, *Acidum nitricum* 30, thrice daily.
(3) With much destruction of tissue, *Kali chlor.* 30, thrice daily.

GINGIVITIS, chronic - See PERIODONTITIS, chronic.

GINGIVITIS of pregnancy
Mercurius sol. 6, twice daily.

GINGIVOSTOMATITIS, acute herpetic (Multiple ulcers of infancy)
(1) With excessive salivation, *Mercurius sol.* 30, thrice daily.
(2) With dry mouth, prostration, drowsiness, *Baptisia* 30, thrice daily.

GUM, diseases of — See ABSCESS, dental; GINGIVITIS, acute ulcerative; GINGIVITIS of pregnancy; GINGIVOSTOMATITIS, acute herpetic; and PERIODONTITIS, chronic.

GUM-BOIL — See ABSCESS, dental.

HAEMATOMA
Arnica 30, thrice daily.

HAEMORRHAGE, dental (acute)
Usually due to extraction, surgery, or accidental oral trauma. Occasionally, due to diseases such as GINGIVITIS, acute ulcerative (q.v.) or leukaemia. When due to extraction, surgery or trauma:
(1) Initially, *Arnica* 200, ¼-hourly.
(2) If bleeding persists, and is bright red, *Ferrum phos.* 30, or *Ipecacuanha* 30, or *Phosphorus* 30, ¼-hourly.
(3) Dark, persistent bleeding, *Lachesis* 30, or *China* 6, hourly.
(4) In haemophiliacs, *Lachesis* 30, ¼-hourly.

HAEMORRHAGE, dental (chronic)
Persistent intermittent bleeding from the gums is usually associated with chronic gingivitis or chronic periodontitis. The latter is a progression of the former, where the periodontal ligament and bone have been attacked by the disease. Loosening of the teeth ensues. (See GINGIVITIS of pregnancy; & PERIODONTITIS, chronic).

HALITOSIS (Offensive breath)
This is usually due to poor oral hygiene, excessive use of tobacco, or the presence of an obvious oral disease, such as GINGIVITIS, acute ulcerative (q.v.). Treatment of these conditions will eliminate halitosis. However, in some instances. the halitosis is not of local origin, but stems from disease of the throat, sinuses, or stomach, which, in turn, are part of a general constitutional problem,

the treatment of which may require the services of a homoeopathic physician. In some cases, the excretion of noxious substances in the breath represents the body's attempt to remove accumulated toxins. To cite an extreme, as in diabetic ketosis. More commonly, the halitosis appears temporarily with detoxifying diets, such as grape cures, juice fasts, and food allergy elimination diets. Where halitosis is not eliminated by the usual dental methods, remedial measures may be attempted before referral to the physician:

(1) *Arnica* 6, twice daily.

(2) *Mercurius sol.* 6, twice daily.

(3) Bad odour from mouth after meals, *Nux vomica* 6, thrice daily.

(4) Mouth covered with offensive mucus after sleep, *Rheum* 6, twice daily.

(5) With constipation, *Acidum carbolicum* 6, twice daily.

(6) With palpitations, *Spigelia* 6, twice daily.

(7) In girls at puberty, *Aurum met.* 6, twice daily.

(8) Like rotten cheese, *Mezereum* 6, twice daily.

(9) Like garlic, *Petroleum* 6, or *Tellurium* 6, twice daily.

(10) Like onions, *Asafoetida* 6, or *Sinapis nigra* 6, twice daily.

(11) Like urine, *Graphites* 6, twice daily.

HERPES LABIALIS (Cold-sores)

(1) In general, for cold-sores and fever blisters, *Natrum mur.* 30, thrice daily.

(2) *Rhus tox.* 30, thrice daily.

(3) Where they are recurrent, constitutional therapy by a homoeopathic physician is required.

INFLUENZA, prevention of

Through their proximity to the patients, dental surgeons have a high risk of contracting this disease. Diminished susceptibility to infection will be gained by:

(1) *Influenzinum Co.* 30, one dose weekly.

(2) Additionally, garlic, garlic and parsley, or odourless garlic tablets/capsules, 1 morning and evening, swallowed with cold water. This will also give a measure of protection against the common cold. Odourless garlic tablets are considered to be less effective than the more usual presentations.

KELOID — See SCAR TISSUE, excessive.

LICHEN PLANUS (lace-like white patches of mouth)

(1) *Arsenicum album* 6, twice daily.

(2) *Natrum phos.* 30, once daily.

LIP, cracked — See also ANGULAR CHEILITIS.

(1) Locally, *Calendula* 5% cream applied sparingly, thrice daily.

(2) Deep crack middle of lower lip, *Natrum mur.* 6, or *Sepia* 6, twice daily.

MORPHOLOGY of teeth, therapeutic relevance of — See CARIES, predisposition to dental.

MOUTH-BREATHING

Frequently due to chronic nasal catarrh and enlarged adenoids in children. In many cases, food allergy is present, and removal of the offending allergen from the diet (most commonly, cow's milk and its products) will produce improvement within a few months. To treat enlarged adenoids (surgery is seldom indicated!):

(1) With much clear mucus, *Agraphis nutans* 6x, twice daily.

(2) In thin children, with pale enlarged tonsils, *Calcarea phosphorica* 30, single doses twice weekly.

(3) In fat children, with cold, clammy feet, *Calcarea carbonica* 30, single doses twice weekly (eg, Mondays and Fridays).

(4) With a family or personal history of tuberculosis, allergy, or asthma, *Tuberculinum Koch* 200, single dose monthly (to be used with caution/supervision in asthma cases).

(5) In children who are always hungry, with sensitive skins, *Sulphur* 30, single dose monthly (to be used with caution/supervision in eczema cases).

(6) In chilly subjects with offensive catarrh, *Psorinum* 30, single dose monthly (caution as with *Sulphur*).

MOUTHWASHES

(1) In general, to reduce pain, swelling and inflammation, infusion of *Salvia offic.* (sage). *Preparation:* Steep one teaspoon of dried or fresh sage leaves in $\frac{1}{2}$ cup of hot water for $\frac{1}{2}$ hour, and strain.

(2) To promote healing, *Calendula lotion. Preparation:* 30 drops ø to 1 pint (500 ml. approx.) water.

(3) To promote healing and reduce pain in aphthous ulcers, *Hydrastis* lotion. *Preparation:* 30 drops ø to $\frac{1}{2}$ pint (250 ml. approx.) water. *These mouthwashes should not be swallowed.*

NEURALGIA, migrainous

The treatment of facial migraine is similar to that of the more classical variety. The constitutional predisposition to this condition often requires therapy from a homoeopathic physician. Since many sufferers have food allergies, improvement may be secured in many instances by elimination of the offending allergen from the diet (most commonly, cow's milk and its products). Treatments for the immediate attack include:

(1) Right-sided neuralgia, *Sanguinaria* 200, $\frac{1}{4}$-hourly.

(2) Left-sided neuralgia, *Spigelia* 200, $\frac{1}{4}$-hourly.

(3) Locally, *Plantago* applied to painful areas of skin or mouth, $\frac{1}{4}$-hourly.

NEURALGIA, Trigeminal (Tic douloureux)

(1) *Aconite* 30, thrice daily.

(2) *Phosphorus* 30, twice daily.

(3) *Verbascum* 30, thrice daily.

(4) *Magnesia phos.* 30, thrice daily.

NOMA (Cancrum oris)

(1) *Mercurius corr.* 6, 2-hourly.

(2) *Kali chlor.* 30, 2-hourly.

(3) Additionally, *Pyrogen* 30, 4-hourly.

ORAL SURGERY, prevention of complications in

Our comments here apply to simple extraction, advanced oral surgery, and periodontal surgery.

(1) Routinely, in all cases, to reduce pain bruising and haemorrhage, *Arnica* 200 and *Hypericum* 30, morning and evening for one day prior to procedure, and seven days after procedure; also a single dose of each, $\frac{1}{2}$ an hour before procedure.

(2) Additionally, where there is a known bleeding tendency, *Phosphorus* 30, in the same dosage.

(3) To prevent infection, add *Pyrogen* 30, twice daily postoperatively for one week.

(4) Locally, to reduce swelling and pain, and promote healing, infusion of *Salvia offic.* mouthwashes, or *Calendula* mouthwashes (see MOUTHWASHES), several times daily postoperatively.

(5) To prevent chest complications from general anaesthesia in chesty patients, add *Antimonium tart.* 6, thrice daily for several days before, and one week after procedure.

(6) To arouse patient after general anaesthesia, *Opium* 30 (drops) $\frac{1}{4}$-hourly. (See also SUBACUTE BACTERIAL ENDOCARDITIS, prevention of.)

ORAL SURGERY, nerve damage from

To promote regeneration of nerve tissue, *Hypericum* 6 twice daily.

ORTHODONTICS

To assist in the repair of the periodontal tissues, *Ruta* 6, twice daily.

OSTEOMA — See TUMOURS & CYSTS.

OSTEOMYELITIS of mandible

(1) *Phosphorus* 30, 4-hourly.

(2) *Hekla lava* 6x, 4-hourly.

(3) *Amphisboena* 30, 4-hourly.

(4) Additionally, *Pyrogen* 30, twice daily.

PAIN THRESHOLD, low

Chamomilla 200, one hour prior to procedure, and repeated $\frac{1}{4}$-hourly as necessary.

PALSY, Bell's
(1) Initially, *Aconite* 30, 2-hourly.
(2) If it fails to respond, then *Causticum* 30, 2-hourly.
(3) After these, *Kali chlor.* 30, 4-hourly.

PARALYSIS, non-cerebral facial — See PALSY, Bell's; & ORAL SURGERY, nerve damage from.

PERICORONITIS (Inflammation around wisdom tooth)
(1) Locally, mouthwashes of infusion of *Salvia offic.* (See MOUTHWASHES), several times daily.
(2) With much throbbing, *Belladonna* 30, 2-hourly.
(3) To promote expulsion of pus, *Hepar sulph.* 6, thrice daily.

PERIODONTAL SURGERY — See ORAL SURGERY, prevention of complications in.

PERIODONTITIS, acute traumatic (Blow to tooth)
Arnica 200 and *Ruta* 30, 4-hourly.

PERIODONTITIS, chronic (Pyorrhoea) —See HAEMORRHAGE, dental (chronic).
In addition to the more usual periodontic procedures, homoeopathic remedies can reduce the severity of the condition, and its rate of progression.
(1) Bleeding gums, foul breath, tongue large and retains imprint of teeth, *Mercurius sol.* 6, once daily.
(2) Bleeding gums, great loss of periodontal bone, "periodontosis", *Phosphorus* 6, once daily.
(3) For control of tartar, see CALCULUS, dental (See also DIET).

PUNCTURE WOUND from instrument
(1) *Ledum* 30, thrice daily.
(2) Additionally, where septicaemia threatens, *Pyrogen* 30, thrice daily.

PYORRHOEA — See PERIODONTITIS, chronic.

RANULA
(1) *Thuja* 6, once daily.
(2) *Mercurius sol.* 6, once daily (may be used in alternation with *Thuja*).

SALIVATION, excessive
(1) Salivation accompanying nervous headache, *Iris vers.* 30, 2-hourly.
(2) Copious salivation after eating, *Allium sativum* 6, thrice daily.
(3) Saliva runs out in sleep, *Baryta carb.* 30, twice daily.
(4) May accompany various obvious oral disorders such as GINGIVITIS, acute

ulcerative, or GINGIVITIS of pregnancy (q.v.). Also seen in Mercury toxicity.

SALIVATION, diminished
Accompanies dehydration, sun-stroke, and febrile illness. Additionally:
(1) Dry mouth with no thirst, *Pulsatilla* 6, twice daily.
(2) Very dry mouth, with dryness of all mucous membranes, great thirst, *Bryonia* 6, twice daily.

SCALDS — See BURNS, instrument.

SCALING & POLISHING, sore gums after
(1) Locally, mouthwashes of *Salvia offic.* infusion, or *Calendula* lotion (see MOUTHWASHES), several times daily.
(2) *Arnica* 30, 2-hourly.

SCAR TISSUE, excessive
(1) Keloid scars of skin, *Graphites* 6, twice daily, plus local application of *Graphites* 8x cream twice daily to scar.
(2) To prevent excessive scar tissue formation after intraoral operations, *Thiosinaminum* 6, twice daily.

SIMILIMUM
The most appropriate remedy for the treatment of a particular patient. The best matched remedy.

SOCKET, infected — See DRY SOCKET.

STOMATITIS
Inflammation of the oral mucosa. (See APHTHOUS ULCERS; GINGIVITIS, ulcerative; GINGIVOSTOMATITIS, acute herpetic; & NOMA.)

STONE — See CALCULUS, salivary.

SUBACUTE BACTERIAL ENDOCARDITIS, prevention of
Pyrogen 30, twice daily, for one day prior to, and up to seven days after procedure.

TASTE, diminished or lost
(1) Complete loss of taste, *Natrum mur.* 6, or *Magnesia carb.* 6, twice daily.
(2) Taste and smell lost after a cold, *Magnesia mur.* 6, thrice daily.
(3) Loss of taste, with thick white coating of tongue, *Antimonium crud.* 6, thrice daily.
(4) Food seems tasteless, milky coating of tongue, *Antimonium tart.* 6, thrice daily.

TASTE, mutated
(1) Food tastes bitter, *Natrum mur.* 6, or *China* 6, or *Pulsatilla* 6, twice daily.
(2) Bread tastes sweet, *Mercurius sol.* 6, twice daily.
(3) Everything tastes salty, *Belladonna* 6, thrice daily.
(4) Food tastes sour, *Nux vomica* 6, or *Lycopodium* 6, twice daily.
(5) Taste of food lingers after eating, *Natrum mur.* 6, or *Acidum nitricum* 6, twice daily.
(6) Food tastes peppery, *Hydrastis* 6, thrice daily.

TASTE, illusions of
(1) Bad taste after sleeping, *Nux vomica,* 6, or *Rheum* 6, twice daily.
(2) Bitter taste, though normal whilst eating, *Chelidonium* 6, twice daily.
(3) Metallic taste, *Cuprum met.* 6, or *Aesculus hip.* 6, or *Mercurius sol.* 6, twice daily.

TEETHING, constitutional upsets in
(1) Child very fractious, whining restlessness, tearful, wishes to be carried or petted, and better for it, may have diarrhoea, *Chamomilla* 30, hourly as necessary (the major remedy).
(2) Similar to previous type, but whole child smells sour, sour diarrhoea, *Rheum* 30, hourly as necessary.
(3) Excessive salivation, sore gums, foul breath, diarrhoea, *Mercurius sol.* 6, twice daily.

TEMPOROMANDIBULAR JOINT, disorders of
(1) Cracking of the joint, *Rhus tox.* 30, twice daily.
(2) Painful cracking of the joint, *Granatum* 6, thrice daily.
(3) Pain in joint on swallowing, *Arum triph.* 30, twice daily.
(4) Joint easily dislocated, *Petroleum* 6, twice daily. (See also FRACTURE, jaw).

TENNIS ELBOW of dentists
Ruta 6, thrice daily.

THRUSH, oral
(1) *Borax* 30, thrice daily (the major remedy).
(2) *Kali mur.* 6x, 4-hourly.
(3) *Natrum mur.* 6x, 4-hourly.
(4) If persistent, *Psorinum* 30, once daily (to be used with caution/supervision in eczema cases).

TONGUE, burning sensation of
In some cases this signifies Vitamin B12, Vitamin B2, or Vitamin B6 deficiency, and replacement therapy will cure. In many other cases, however, the

cause is more obscure. Remedies include:

(1) *Arsenicum album* 6, twice daily.

(2) *Ignatia* 6, twice daily.

(3) *Iris vers.* 6, twice daily. Problematical cases should be referred to a homoeopathic physician.

TOOTH-GRINDING/CLENCHING — See BRUXISM, BRUXOMANIA.

TOOTHACHE

Where the pain is related to ABSCESS, dental; NEURALGIA, migrainous; NEURALGIA, trigeminal; PERICORONITIS, etc., treat as indicated in appropriate section. Otherwise:

(1) *Plantago* 6, ¼-hourly (the first remedy).

(2) In association with many black stumps, *Staphysagria* 30, hourly.

(3) Pain utterly intolerable, *Chamomilla* 200, ½-hourly.

(4) Toothache in pregnancy, *Sepia* 6, 4-hourly.

(5) Locally, *Plantago* ø applied to painful area of mouth, ¼-hourly.

TRISMUS

Reflex spasm of the jaw muscles is a concomitant feature of many oral conditions such as ABSCESS, dental; and BRUXISM, BRUXOMANIA (q.v.). Treatment should proceed along the lines indicated. Rarely, it is caused by tetanus.

TUMOURS & CYSTS — See also RANULA.

(1) Cysts and tumours of the jaws causing bony expansion, *Hekla lava* 6x, twice daily.

(2) Osteoma, *Calcarea fluorica* 30, twice weekly.

(3) Haemangioma, *Calcarea fluorica* 30, twice weekly.

(4) For the treatment of oral malignancy; alternative treatment is available in the forms of dietetic modification, the application of homoeopathic remedies, and the use of injections of *Viscum album* to stimulate the immune response against the cancer. Referral to a homoeopathic physician is necessary.

ULCERS, common mouth — See APHTHOUS ULCERS.

ULCERS of infancy — See GINGIVOSTOMATITIS, acute herpetic.

VINCENT'S STOMATITIS — See GINGIVITIS, acute ulcerative.

WISDOM TOOTH, inflammation around — See PERICORONITIS.

WRIST of dentist, sprained
Ruta 6, thrice daily.